Contents

Health Hacks:

46 *Hacks* to Improve Your Mood, Boost Your Performance, and Guarantee a Longer, Healthier, More Vibrant Life

By C.K. Murray

Chances are, you're like me.

Human. And if you're human, you're tired. You're tired of the bullshit; tired of people telling you to do this and to do that, tired and frustrated of all the hula-hoops you jump through over and over just to make ends meet.

"It's got to be easier than this," you think. Because at the end of the day, *this* simply ain't cuttin' it.

If you've ever watched a movie featuring computers, you've probably heard of hacking. In a nutshell, hacking is a way to cut through the fluff. It might not be the prettiest route to success, and it certainly isn't the nicest, but it is *by far* the easiest. And the quickest.

Assuming you know what you're doing...

See, when we picture hacking and hackers, certain images seem to dominate. Maybe we imagine a dude in a dark basement, surrounded by cryptic computer screens and empty Redbull cans, feverishly typing his way into the FBI mainframe. Or maybe we picture a group of devious teenagers, with their genius IQs and directionless futures, stealing credit card info with the click of a mouse.

No matter who you are or what you do, hacking can benefit your life.

But wait…

What is "Health Hacking"?

Good question, dear reader, and I thank you for asking.

Basically, it doesn't matter what your position or trajectory in life may be, whether you're a part-time worker, a careerist, or currently unemployed—understanding health hacking is essential. By hitting the right buttons, we literally dictate how we feel, how we look, how we think and how we perform. And when these everyday capabilities become stronger, healthier, and more vibrant, there is nowhere to go but *up*.

Health hacking is about taking the same mentality that optimizes computing, and using it on our minds and bodies. When we health hack, we get to the root of good health and we get there fast.

Let's face it, most of us don't have the time or resources to completely overhaul our lives. Although so-called experts may scream at us to undergo massive lifestyle changes, it simply ain't gonna happen. We've got commitments, and jobs and plans and planners and paper lists of things to-do that we're so far behind on, we feel as if the weight of the world is pressing on our chest.

Some of us simply don't have the capability to make comprehensive changes right away.

And this is where health hacking comes into play. Think about it. What if you can bypass all the legwork? What if you can hit all the right buttons when you *want* to?

Want to clear your skin? Want to boost your thinking power? Looking to get in better cardiovascular shape? Hoping to shave a few pounds and attract that coveted partner? Want nothing more than to feel happier and healthier? To look and feel more confident?

Good, you get the picture. Now let's get right down to it. It's time to hack.

In the following pages, you will learn a variety of powerful and easy shortcuts to physical and mental health. These hacks are not always mainstream, and some of them will leave you shocked. Your doctor won't readily recommend these strategies, and you're probably not going to stumble across them in the majority of the literature.

But remember, these health hacks are designed to bypass the 'norm.' They're unconventional, and in some cases, counterintuitive.

Still, that doesn't make them wrong.

None of the following hacks are nonsense. It's all scientifically proven, and it's all scientifically proven to boost your health today. Not next month, not a year from now. TODAY. We're talking about immediate gains here.

But enough with the pep talk, let's get down to the goods.

Chew Away the Fat

What if you could actually curb your appetite, shed pounds and leave the cravings behind by chewing?

That's right, we're talking about gum here. So grab your favorite flavor, freshen your breath and kill your appetite. Several studies have shown that chewing gum after lunch can lower the appetite by as much as 10%. In other words, people consumed 10% less snacks than those who did not. Gum chewing stimulates eating motions such as taste, jaw movement, salivation and swallowing. You trick your brain and stomach into thinking you're eating when you're not! Not to mention, gum chewing will also stimulate a certain level of relaxation.

This may be why gum-chewers tend to score higher on the SATs! Just be careful: if you're chewing a lot, choose gum that isn't too sugary. And don't chew too vigorously, unless you're trying to build up a bulky jaw.

The Ultimate Sugar Substitute

Forget the Splenda and the artificial replacements. Cinnamon is flavorful and low in calories. It comes from Asia and is a great substitute for sugar on and in many of our favorite drinks and foods. For starters, throw it in your cup of coffee and forego the overload of sugar. Say goodbye to sugar crashes and diabetes, and say hello to the numerous health benefits of cinnamon. That's right, this lovely spice has been shown to have "anti-inflammatory, antimicrobial, antioxidant, antitumor, cardiovascular, cholesterol-lowering, and immunomodulatory effects."

Spice it up!

Liquid Metabolism

Water is everywhere, and we're not taking advantage of it. Hook yourself up to the mainline and take advantage!

Water leads to weight loss and actually accelerates metabolism. It is a great general health strategy as well as a way to improve athletic fitness. Water is so critical to our bodies and our brains, but many of us are uninformed. Not to mention, *most* of us are chronically dehydrated. The effects of water are truly remarkable.

If you don't like normal water due to its blandness, spice it up with fruit infusion recipes! Also, feel free to gain water from the following foods: watermelon, cucumber, strawberries, celery, coconut water, soup, and even coffee.

Cool—don't burn—the fat off!

The best way to lose weight without actually doing anything is to set the temperature right. Studies have shown that people who sleep in cool rooms are significantly more likely to develop what's known as 'brown fat.' Brown fat is actually more muscle than fat, meaning that it burns off other unseemly fats and actually boosts the metabolic rate. 66-degrees is considered the ideal temperature. You can also do this in your home or workplace, all the time. Once your body adjusts to the slightly lower temperature, you'll be fine. Try to wear nothing but light pajamas and bed sheets at night.

One study showed that people doubled their percentage of brown fat, and were burning more calories throughout the waking hours.

Armpit Garnish

Lemons are great due to their super amount of vitamin C. They are also great because they can freshen almost everything stored nearby in your kitchen. This is because the citric acid helps to slow oxidation, thus delaying browning. However, you probably didn't know that lemon juice is also a great last-minute deodorant replacement.

Simply shoot some on your smelly spots and go about your business. Lemon juice mixed with 2/3 water can also highlight your hair. Oh, and it can also be used to ward of mosquitoes and bugs when sprayed or added to door and window crevices. Pretty handy, eh?

Less L Bsss, More Z Z Zsss

We all know that sleep is important, but who knew that not getting enough will actually keep us heavier? See, when we lack sleep, our metabolism goes down as our brains' secretion of cortisol gets out of whack. Cortisol is the hormone associated with stress, and when we're stressed our body is not very adept at keeping weight regulated. Not to mention, having broken or interrupted sleep can also drastically impact our health.

Sleep more , weigh less!

Don't "Diet." Diet!

Research shows that diet soda is actually a major culprit in weight gain. Although many people buy diet for its alleged health benefits, contrary to sugar, this is simply not true. Artificial sweeteners activate our brains in strange ways, causing an addiction to an unhealthy beverage additive. Basically, avoid diet soda just as you would any other sugary drink.

Instead, enjoy some infused water!

Less is More and More is Less

That is to say, when it comes to eating, less is more. Try to eat 5-6 meals a day, with each meal being smaller than if you were to shove down two or three a day. This Is good because it keeps your metabolism chugging and doesn't stagnate you with oversized helpings. Your body is designed to receive constant small amounts of fuel. Throwing a ton of logs on the fire once or twice a day is much less efficient than feeding the flames smaller sticks throughout the day.

Not to mention, all this constant small-sized eating will tempt you from binging or eating less healthy foods. Try snacks such as bananas, apples, whole wheat bread, hummus, and others.

Drink the Ocean

Not literally, but kinda.

See, sea salt is actually good for you. And all you need is a little—just 1/16th of a teaspoon for an 8oz glass of water. Add it in to facilitate hydration. This is good because it helps our bodies run more seamlessly. Most of the time, we just chug water, but water alone won't hydrate us completely.

Sea salt is the answer. It is a natural salt that provides 80 trace minerals in a form that our body can use readily. It boosts blood sugar, strengthens bones, steadies metabolism, and jacks up the immune system, among many other benefits.

Creating a 'Museum of Memories'

Are you distracted or scatterbrained?

Do you struggle to remember your to-do list? Can't keep track of all the details for work or school or your latest project? Have trouble just keeping a few priorities in order?

Truth be told, the human brain is not good at remembering stuff. At least, stuff that comes on lists. This is the reason we have grocery lists and refrigerator post-its. It's the reason we have itineraries and schedules that we throw on our digital devices for later retrieval.

But what if there was a way to change this?

Just as we can easily remember the location of things—places and destinations—we can also remember our *to-dos* with the same effortless ability. This is because our minds are great at spatial memory. If we can learn to change other important things into a sort of mental environment, then we can remember them too!

Simply associate each item or thing with a specific location. For instance, think about how easy it is to remember places and sights in your neighborhood. You remember certain yards, corner stores, different trees, and cul-de-sacs, and all kinds of manmade and natural sights.

Now, imagine that each location has an item there. Imagine you're driving slowly or walking slowly through your neighborhood streets and roads. In your spatial mind, insert items along the way. The stranger, the better—but it doesn't have to be.

Maybe you see a man cleaning his car at the first crossroads. This reminds you that you intend to clean your own car. Maybe you see a kid raking the leaves at the big house with the blue shutters. So you're reminded that you have yard work on your to-do list. Or maybe you imagine something weird and impossible for the real-world, like an elephant standing outside your local convenience store—a reminder that you want to watch that Animal Channel show coming on next week.

You'll be surprised how effective this technique can be. It's actually one of the 'secrets' of memory champs.

Tart Recovery

Workouts are great for our bodies, but sometimes they leave us sore and stiff as a plank. If you're feeling like you haven't recovered well from your latest blowout, maybe it's time to get tart. That's right, drinking tart cherry juice <u>has been shown</u> to reduce swelling and inflammation once muscles are damaged. This will speed recovery with less pain.

So instead of turning to fancy energy drinks and powders, give a nice tart cherry drink a try. You might wake up feeling loose as a goose!

Carbs are Good!

If you know anything about fiber, you know that it fills you up. Most people need 20-30 grams a day. Fiber is also a carbohydrate, so by eating enough of it, your stomach will feel full and your digestion will thank you. If you have any 'blockages' in the intestinal tract, fiber will help!

Sleep like Superman

Experts are mixed on this one, mainly because it has not been studied in full. Still, some specialists claim that there are many examples and anecdotes showing the benefits of polyphasic sleep. This sleep is said to 'trick' the mind and body into entering only the most crucial portion of sleep, REM sleep.

One of the most common polyphasic sleep schedules is called the Uberman Sleep Schedule, and allows you to maximize waking time while optimizing sleeping time. This schedule is comprised of six 20- to 30-minute power naps every four hours during the day. It's a schedule that can be very tough to get used to, taking weeks sometimes. Still, some experts argue that it is the ideal way to hack your sleeping clock.

Most people adopting this schedule go to bed around 8 p.m., and wake up to the alarm at 8:30. They then go back to bed at midnight and wake up at 12:30. They then continue these intervals indefinitely, struggling with sleep deprivation *at first.*

It is believed that around the week and a half mark, the brain hits a switch that adapts to this superhuman sleeping schedule. Normally people get 90 minutes of REM sleep, considered the most important stage for recovery and healing. It is believed that for those who weather the storm, the brain learns to forego the other stages of sleep and go right into REM sleep.

In this sense, you might be just sitting down for short periods of a time, but every time you do, your mind plunges into REM. In the end, you feel rested and you can spend a lot more time actually awake getting stuff done. Be warned, however, as some disagree. The detractors argue that the Uberman Schedule is not sustainable long-term and can contribute to many health problems associated with sleep deprivation.

Try at your own risk!

Maximize Vitamin Absorption the Natural Way

Although it seems odd, adding in some fats to your vegetables is actually beneficial. Dark leafy greens such as kale, swiss chard, and spinach are well-known for their numerous health benefits. However, these benefits aren't fully realized if we don't take the time to fully absorb the nutrients contained within. If you want to get the most of the fat-soluble vitamins like A, E, and K, you need to eat some dietary fats alongside the vegetables.

For a healthy balance, try to mix them with just a small amount of nuts or a tablespoon or two of olive oil. Just be sure to think out your preparation. Boiling vegetables is common but actually pretty counterproductive. When you're done boiling, you'll see a bunch of colored water. Your best bet is to simply drink that water, since most of the goods in the vegetables have leeched out.

Instead of boiling, try sautéing or even steaming to get the most of your vegetables. This is especially true of carrots, which yield more of their anti-cancer nutrients when cooked as opposed to raw.

Forget the Pill

Probably the most important vitamin out there is Vitamin D. It is both hormone and vitamin, regulating blood pressure, weight, mood, and a bunch of other incredible attributes. Not getting enough Vitamin D has been linked to early heart disease, cancer, softening of the bones, depression, chronic fatigue and an array of other physical and mental health problems.

The good news is, you don't have to buy vitamin pills to get enough of it. All you have to do is get outside and soak up that sun! Just not too much sun, UVB and UVA rays are potentially damaging to the skin.

If you don't spend time outdoors, don't live anywhere near the equator, don't absorb it well due to dark skin, or use sunscreen every time you go out, focus on eating foods fortified with Vitamin D. They are usually labeled as such. Also, try to get out as often as possible! Using a supplement may also help.

The Truth About Egg Yolks

You need to eat them!

Contrary to common belief, egg yolks are not going to lead to coronary heart disease, stroke, or coronary vascular disease. A comprehensive analysis of previous studies found that despite their fat content, whole eggs are good for us.

So don't fret! Heart disease is not caused by saturated fat, but instead by chronic stress, oils and processed foods. If you've been avoiding egg yolks thinking they're bad you've been missing out. You've been missing out on vitamin A, B vitamins for energy, and choline for brain power, muscles, and reproductive health. In fact, the saturated fat in eggs that is said to be so bad is actually good. It helps regulate hormones and the body's absorption of vitamins and minerals.

Eat eggs, just keep them in balance like anything else. And don't load them up with salt. Enjoy them healthily. Capiche?

The T-Factor

Testosterone is not just for men looking to get ripped in the gym. It is a hormone found in both males and females, a hormone that boosts muscle mass, strength, and our brain's capabilities. Without enough testosterone, we store more fat, lose our sex drives, and have an increased risk of cardiovascular disease. Not to mention, premature aging.

The best ways to optimize testosterone are through adequate sleep, balanced diet, and exercise. Saturated fat such as that found in eggs is also good for boosting testosterone levels. Intense exercise such as interval training will also help to spike T. This includes short duration/high intensity runs, pushups, weight exercises, and the like. The testosterone boost can actually be detected in our saliva.

Squash Your Blood Pressure

Summer squash is a great food available year round. Because of its high vitamin C content, summer squash will decrease cortisol levels, reducing stress. It will also give you plenty of B vitamins, which will enable better stress coping. Keep your blood vessels relaxed.

There are numerous other amazing foods for blood pressure too. Combined with magnesium and potassium, these squash constituents will keep you loose and relaxed.

Nature's Smart Drug

It's called peppermint.

It's a member of the mentha species and has been shown to achieve a wide range of benefits. Studies have shown that its aroma alone alleviates stressing perceptions of physical workload, temporal workload, effort, and anxiety. It has also been shown to boost exercise performance and cognitive performance.

Perhaps this is why kids are getting all hopped up on it before standardized tests?

Exam Cram

Do you have a huge exam, assessment, or work-related project coming up? Have you been procrastinating, fretting, and thinking that there's *no way* you'll get it all done?

Well, turns out cramming is not the way to go. Although some may swear by their ability to shove all the information in their brain and then spew it out while it's still fresh, this strategy actually goes against everything we know about memory. See, the human brain retains information through the process of acquisition, consolidation, and recall. And we only fully consolidate information while we sleep.

When you sleep, your brain works its neural connections and integrates what you learned awake. Thus, it's no surprise that a lot of research shows that people perform better on cognitive tests after a 24-hr period including sleep. Those who test after cramming just 20-30 minutes earlier, perform the worst .

Immune Vision

Research shows that mere images can boost our immune systems. Just as your mind and body may react to sexual imagery or pleasant imagery or violent imagery, your body also reacts to images of unhealthiness. Studies show that when people have to look at images of disgusting infections, health problems, or injuries, their bodies actually undergo chemical changes. The immune system will send its white blood cells into production, pumping out a protein known to combat infection.

This has an evolutionary reason. When we see people in real-life who look sick, our brain tells our body to get on its horse and beef up its defense. It's a natural way to prevent us from contracting whatever they have. Perhaps this may help explain why so many physicians don't get sick despite being around patients all the time. Not only are physician immune systems bolstered by constant exposure to patients, but those immune systems are also bolstered simply by *seeing* those patients.

Meatless Protein

You don't need to eat meat if you don't want to. For those foregoing meat due to vegetarianism or veganism, or for some other reason (such as religion), legumes are a good alternative. Legumes include beans, chickpeas and lentils.

They can be soaked and cooked, included in chili, salads, tacos, or by themselves. Because the CDC recommends getting as much as 35% of our calories in protein, it's important to take this seriously—especially if we don't eat meat.

The good news is, legumes can be found in most grocery stores in the dried and canned goods sections. They're not expensive and they're pretty versatile. So enjoy!

Sinus Relief Now!

Instead of experimenting with weird sprays and allergy medicines that make you drowsy, give this one a try: chop up an onion, throw it all in a bowl and suck in those powerful fumes. This will relieve congestion and pressure pretty easily.

Green Skin for the Win

Avocado is delicious. It's also very versatile. You can enjoy it in tacos and burritos, you can use it as a substitute for butter, in tuna and chicken salads as a substitute for mayo, and even cooked with an egg in the middle (once the pit is removed).

But did you know that avocado is also great for your skin? It is—so drop the expensive exfoliators. If you want the generous helping of vitamins E and B6 contained in every avocado, simply mash down the fruit and slather it on. It might seem odd at first, but your skin will love you for it!

The Sweetest Solution

The research doesn't lie.

If you want a quick burst of energy, forget 5-hour or some pricey gel. Instead, opt for one or two spoonfuls of honey. Honey's powerful natural sugars are just as effective, and will carry you through most endurance exercises. Great before, during or after a run or hike.

But the beauty of honey doesn't stop there. It is also a natural cough suppressant, lip balm, and moisturizer. Don't give it to children under age 1 for coughs, but otherwise use it like you would cough syrup. Take a couple spoonfuls and feel better! For lips, rub on a little to protect against dryness. And for dry skin, rub in and leave for half an hour. Just be sure to wash away—and don't overdo, lest you get too sticky.

Shampoo Alternatives

Dry hair, split ends, damaged hair and thinning hair are embarrassing and unseemly. Blow dryers, curling irons and flat irons all contribute to poor hair health, but if you can't get away from these products try olive oil. The fatty acids in olive oil protect hair by making it more soft and controllable. All you have to do is leave it in for 10 minutes or so and then rinse out. The hair will be shinier too.

Lemon and beer also help. The hops in beer soothe hair while half a lemon's worth of juice combined with water will help clear up dandruff. Let it sit in the hair for 10 minutes or so before rinsing thoroughly.

Most shampoos are scented with these natural ingredients, but also contain other potentially harmful chemicals, such as some surfactants. Forego these foreign agents and let your hair bask in its newfound, all-natural glory!

Hiccup Hack

Who *isn't* annoyed by hiccups?

One moment you're sitting there fine, the next moment you sound like you belong in a pigsty. If you've tried everything to cure your hiccups, from getting scared to holding your breath, try this:

Down a teaspoon of raw honey or coconut sugar (organic). Because hiccups are caused by diaphragm spasms, it is believed that the honey and sugar soothe the nerve muscles. This relaxation is a nice way to feel better instantly.

Blow Anxiety Away

We all get nervous. Whether fretting a first date, hoping for a good presentation, or anticipating a medical procedure, there are a million different ways to get nervous and anxious.

But there's an easy way to ease the tension. Before you pop a valium, try blowing your thumb. That's right, blow your thumb. The thumb is said to have its own pulse and blowing on it will cool down that area and that pulse. Also, breathing in deep for a blow naturally calms your heart.

Deep breaths and cool air. Who woulda thunk?

Brain Loops

Turns out, doodling is actually quite productive!

If you've ever been thinking deeply, daydreaming, or vaguely considering an idea, you might have found yourself lazily drawing stuff in the margins. Many times, this 'stuff' may turn out to be squiggles, faces, shapes, diamonds, or some hybrid of it all.

However, research shows that what really matters is the drawing itself. When researchers asked a group of participants to trace two different styles, they found some surprising results. The group asked to trace jagged lines differed on a later creative test from the group asked to trace elegant, looping lines.

The reasoning behind this is that looping lines are most favorable. They mimic the fluid and unrestricted nature of the human brain, which doesn't like to be fitted into jagged modes of thinking. It is also more relaxing and allows the 'natural juices' to flow freely.

Sunburn Healing

If you don't have aloe Vera or some other miracle cure, tea is a good home remedy. What you need is to acquire a pitcher and several bags of black tea. Make sure the water is lukewarm in the pitcher and allow the teabags to soak until the water is pitch black. Then, soak a rag in this tea water and drape it over the burned area. This will soothe the flesh and accelerate the recovery.

The Fruit That Cleans Teeth!

Do you like apples?

Well you should! Apples are great not only for their rich nutritional content, but also because of the process involved in eating them. A solid, crunchy apple removes excess food and bacteria as you chew. Apples also have what is known as malic acid, which helps dissolve stains. In fact, malic acid is actually used in many teeth-whitening products!

Hack your Head

This refers to two specific phenomenon that originate in your head: brainfreeze and headache. For brainfreezes, press the tongue flat against the roof of the mouth. The more area you can cover, the better. When the nerves at the roof of the mouth get cold, your head overheats as compensation, causing that unique pain of the brainfreeze. The tongue on the roof helps end that temperature disparity. For actual headaches, take the thumb and forefinger and pinch down on the muscle on the web of your other hand, holding for a couple minutes. This is considered a shiatsu point and is believed to ease the headache by stimulating blood flow. Unfortunately, this has not been researched in-depth, and its effectiveness is mostly anecdotal and mystical.

Going 'Mad Men'

If you've ever seen the show, you get the idea. Basically, going 'mad men' means getting drunk. Sloshed. Hammered at work.

Although most people would caution against such libation, studies show that a little alcohol has nice effects on workplace productivity. Or shall we say, ingenuity. In fact, alcohol has been shown to spark creative ideas at the cost of diminishing focus. Basically, you can't focus as well because your brain jumps all over the place; but in doing so, it increases the idea of innovative solutions. Or, at the very least, the start of an innovation solution…

Not many studies have targeted this phenomenon, but one such piece of research is especially illuminating. When brought to a BAC of .075, participants solved more Remote Associates Test items more quickly than their sober counterparts. The result of this study shed light on the fascinating nature of memory, working memory especially.

Having a great working memory means that an individual is good at screening out extraneous information. This is good for analytical problems, but bad for tangential or diffusive issues. When alcohol (and drugs too) expand our awareness in their unique ways, we are less likely to think systematically and incrementally, and more likely to come to thoughts in leaps and bounds.

Just don't get too drunk. You don't want to go leaping or bounding off the wrong ledge…

Hack the Gag

One in three people don't have a gag reflex. But for the rest of us normal suckers, the pharyngeal relax can be a real gag. I mean.. drag.

It happens when the muscles in our throat contract due to a certain penetration or aversive visual stimulus like vomit. Fortunately, there is more than one good way to fight the reflex. Research indicates that by pressing a point on the palm or by squeezing your thumb in a fist, you can effectively cut off the muscle contraction that would occur.

So stop gagging. Stop choking. Feel better at the dentist, feel better brushing your teeth, feel better with whatever odd objects you enjoy plunging in there…

Allergic to Weight Loss

Turns out those lovely little meds you take for your runny nose and itchy skin are keeping you heavier. Studies show that people on antihistamines are ten pounds heavier on average than their unmedicated counterparts, due to the fact that antihistamines prevent histamines from playing their regular role in fat breakdown. So next time you reach for the Allegra or Claritin, consider the alternative: corticosteroids, allergy shots, or simply a diet and exercise adjustment.

Peanut Butter Shave

That's right, baby. Shave your skin with peanut butter (the creamier, the better). The natural oils help to keep the skin fresh and moist, leaving behind a pretty interesting scent.

Just don't lick it! Well, not in public at least…

The Angry Hand

There's always that one person who loses his or her temper way too easily. For people like this, or simply for people looking to practice self-control, consider this: the key to less anger is in your hand. Increased self-control doesn't come from calming images or pleasing mantras, as much as it comes from using the right hand.

Which hand is the right hand, you ask? Well, it depends.

For most people, the correct hand to use is the left hand. In other words, use your non-dominant hand. Research shows that using your non-dominant hand for virtually all nonviolent tasks will lead to diminished activity in the areas of the brain associated with lack of self-control. In other words, use your weak hand and you'll get so used to minor struggles, that you'll become more calm about things that would normally set you off. That is, if you can last long enough to see the results (roughly 2 weeks).

Uncomfortably Creative

We like to think that problem-solving occurs best under optimal conditions. That is to say, we assume that the more comfortable and confident we are with ourselves or others, the more likely we are to work well together and produce great results. For this reason, morning people will attempt difficult tasks in the morning, and night-owls late at night.

But this is not supported by the science. Research shows you actually accomplish the most creative solutions if you do them when you think you're at your worst. You are less at ease and more inclined to thinking outside the box. If you do things when you're comfortable, around others with whom you are comfortable, you think more normally.

So throw yourself into dangerous waters, and force yourself to do what you don't want to. Your brain might just respond with brilliance.

The Energy Rub

Before you reach for another coffee, Redbull, or Five Hour Energy, consider this: the self-massage. But not just any massage. To stimulate your body and mind, you need to tap into the wherewithal of ancient Chinese medicine.

Massage your ears! By stimulating the pressure points in the ears, we successfully increase blood circulation to the whole body.

Energy, here I come.

Sedentary Garlic

Garlic is widely used. It's a nice addition to many dishes and appetizers, adding a depth of flavor and a variety of great health benefits. The only problem is, the *vast* majority of people prepare it the wrong way.

DO NOT throw your garlic into the heated pan right off the bat. DO NOT

The protein element called alliin and the heat-modulated enzyme alliinase are the key constituents at work here. These two properties synthesize when we cut garlic, but only if given time. If we throw them right to the flames, the cancer-fighting, heart-strengthening properties disappear. But if we wait 10 minutes, they fully coalesce, and then the balance is right. And they will stay that way through the entire cooking process!

Hydration Hack Points

Yea, yea, we all know that water is necessary for hydration. The real question is: when's the best time to drink it?

Firstly, drink to start off your day, to get your organs going. Then, make sure to drink half an hour before every meal to facilitate digestion and absorption. Then, drink before taking a bath to lower your blood pressure. And finally, be sure to drink before going to bed—to stave of strokes and heart attacks.

Face your Feelings. Literally

They say not to judge a book by its cover, but let's be honest. We all do it.

We also all judge a face by its features. And we *all* judge a person's mood by those features, and expressions. As it turns out, science has a reason for this. When we smile, our brain likes to get feedback from our muscles before telling us how we feel. In this sense, simply smiling can make us feel happier, just as simply frowning can make us feel sadder. Our facial muscles are directly tied to the release of hormones in our brains and bodies.

This is supported by other research that shows the power of Botox. This well-known cosmetic drug is used to paralyze muscles, believed to relieve creases and lines in the flesh. However, by paralyzing the facial muscles and rendering a display of emotion almost impossible, the brain also feels rather emotionless.

In one critical study, researchers exposed people who had recently received Botox to emotionally-charged videos. The participants exhibited few biological responses and reported feeling few as well. Those who did not receive Botox were strongly affected.

Caffeinated Power Naps

This probably sounds like a conundrum.

How the heck can one take a nap after ingesting caffeine? While it's true that some people are so desensitized to caffeine, they can down a latte and go right to sleep, most of us do not have this superpower. However, most of us have not fully considered the tactic.

See, caffeine takes effect after roughly 15 minutes and isn't ingested till 45 in. This means that you can drink a cup of joe, grab a quick 15 minute nap, and wake up with the caffeine surge hitting its full stride. If you're exhausted and can fall asleep quickly, this tactic will work wonders. You'll get both the nice effects of a power nap and the energy boost of your favorite upper.

BOOM, BABY!

Eat Away Your Cramp

Cramps suck, but what if they're caused by something simple?

Studies show that many cramps and aches, especially in the legs, can be the result of potassium deficiency. What's rich in potassium, you ask?

Bananas! Oh, and just to be safe, make sure you're well-hydrated. Dehydration is also a common cause of cramps, Charlie-horses, and other muscles spasms and problems.

Teabaggin' It

Tea has long been touted for its numerous health benefits. But did you know that it is also a major player in healthy weight maintenance? One of green tea's main antioxidants can up our metabolic rate for an entire day. We should seek to drink two or three cups a day, but only if they're coming from a rich source of tea such as Teavana Gyokuro Imperial Green Tea.

Get the benefits now!

Allergy Hacks

Allergies are a pain the ass, and we've all experienced them to one degree or another.

But did you know that allergies can be treated almost entirely without medication? That's right, all it takes is the right approach and some gradual exposure, and you're well on your way to sneeze-free, itch-free days.

Eating quality honey is one way to do it. Just as allergists will administer allergy shots in what is called 'immunotherapy,' eating honey every day is a similar approach. Honey is full of the very pollen spores that make life tough for seasonal allergy sufferers. By exposing the body's immune system to small amounts of honey, we become acclimated to these pesky allergens, and our bodies learn to decrease the production of responding histamines. The concentration in honey is low enough so that it doesn't cause our antibodies to trigger allergic reactions. Over time, we can up the amount of honey we consume, but the most important part is to consume it regularly. Also, be sure that the honey consumed is local, high-quality honey. You want as much of that natural as possible, so look in a health food store or farmer's market.

You've probably heard of other approaches like humidifiers and tea, but what you really want to do is treat the source. These problems will alleviate the symptoms, but the main goal should be to stop those symptoms from ever occurring. That means building antibodies and bolstering the immune system. It's a more gradual process, but will save you a lot of headaches (literally) and a lot of money.

Another way to achieve this is by eliminating foods known to induce allergic reactions such as peanuts, eggs, dairy, wheat, fish, shellfish, and soy. It will be hard at first, but after a few weeks you will likely start to see a difference in your symptoms.

Now, this is where the acclimation comes into play. Slowly reintroduce each food group, one by one. Take a week or two for each reintroduction. Start by eating just a few pieces of fish here and there, then slowly pick up the habit. See, all of these food groups are great for us when consumed in balance. If they are triggering allergic reactions, we want to build our immune system up to them—just as we did with the honey.

It's also important to gauge which food type is giving you the most problems. If you feel really crummy after wheat but not eggs, remove the wheat and try to acclimate fully to eggs before reintroducing the wheat later. All of this is based on a theory that exposure to small amounts of harmful things is ultimately good for us. It's called 'hormesis.'

It's also the reason that doctors are discovering that many sickly children live in homes that are over-sanitized. This occurs because the parents of these children go to great lengths to spray cleaners and air fresheners all throughout the house, thus eliminating bacteria and germs. The only problem is, the homes are so clean, that growing children never adapt to certain bacteria, leading to compromised immune systems and likely allergy problems down the road.

As with everything in life, balance is key. You don't want to eliminate all the germs . It will only end up hurting you in the end.

So now you know. Health hacking is about taking shortcuts, using things you never thought were possible, and boosting your life to all new levels. Instead of relying on heavy doses of medicine or complicated physician visits, health hacking makes it simple. You will think clearer, you will feel stronger, you will and look and perform better than ever!

So stop what you're doing. Stop trying to make it through in the same old boring way. Stop trying to be normal like everybody else. It's time to bypass the bullshit and get straight to the source. Don't waste time, don't squander your resources.

Hack Your Health TODAY!

A Special Note:

Thank you for reading *"Health Hacks: 46 Hacks to Improve Your Mood, Boost Your Performance, and Guarantee a Longer, Healthier, More Vibrant Life."* If you enjoyed reading this book and would like to be included on an email list for when similar content is available, feel free:

Sign-Up Now

As always, thank you for reading.

And may you continue to live healthily and happily.

Sincerely,

C.K. Murray

Other works by C.K. Murray:

www.ingramcontent.com/pod-product-compliance
Lightning Source LLC
Chambersburg PA
CBHW070613290526
45790CB00002B/903